CHRISTINE ALLEN

THE FEET I HAVE FELT

A catalogue record for this work is available from the National Library of Australia

NATIONAL LIBRARY OF AUSTRALIA

National Library of Australia Catalogue-in-Publication data:

The Feet I Have Felt/Christine Allen

ISBN:
978-1-7636406-8-9
(Paperback)

My book is dedicated to the late Lord Erne of Crom who initially prompted me to write about the feet i have felt.

To my late best friend Hazel Johston who told me in a dream to get it finished.

INTRODUCTION

Christine Allen is sharing a different view on health from her own experiences over the last 40 years. She has had great success through a wealth of experience working daily on people with the help of reflexology and homeopathy.

'A gift from higher levels'

I do believe, as many have said, in 'a gift from higher levels'. This I did not accept until well into my years of practice. I was born on 20 December 1961 to parents Sean and Marie McCourt in County Tyrone, Northern Ireland. My mother was a nurse with a very physical knowledge outside her hospital duties which I used to admire greatly and thought how can she tell that she is not a doctor but was always correct in her assessment, so I believe today she has passed that on to me.

As a young 9/10 years old I was crippled with leg problems and walked and hopped along, unable to run and play my favourite games, hopscotch and tennis, and was brought to many orthopaedic surgeons – all in vain.

Until one day when I started doing my practical training for chiropody and I discovered my saviour Walter Hynes. He finished up every day with his treatments, pulled back a curtain and there stood a long black couch.

Now he said: 'Christine, give me another occupation I practice. I'm one of a kind.' And so he was.

It was reflexology, a word I had never heard of. He started working on the feet, and I clearly remember him working on an amputee one day. I thought this strange as he obviously only had one foot. 'Oh,' he said, 'but he has two hands, so right foot and left hand.'

All very intriguing.

I have to learn how to do this.

'Well,' he said, 'England or Cork is where you will have to go.' And so my journey started.

Going back to my 8- and 9-year-old self, I was a very mischievous child. I couldn't play on the playground, but my school was beside the local church, so I decided to do a little bit of acting. Dressing up in the priest robes pretending to say mass. Oops! In walked the local sexton.

And in his bruff loud voice let one unmerciful roar at me: 'What are you at? Your parents will hear about this.'

The class of my friends scurried like mice out through the back door of the church and left me standing in my green and white robes.

At the age of 11 I got knocked down by a taxi on my way to music lessons. Obviously, years later I became the organist for evening prayer on Sundays. I moved to grammar school. The convent in Omagh, and again these devilish tendencies came back. I was at it again: dressing up and mimicking. Caught again by the head sister Barbara, we bargained so I had to join the school choir. My love for music saved me.

The day Elvis died

These attributes I carried on into my work. When I was 16, I travelled to Canada on my own to meet cousins I have never seen in my 16 years of living. It was the day Elvis Presley died. The family (Tasker was their name) were more traumatised about Elvis rather than meeting their long-lost cousin. From there I travelled on the Greyhound Bus for 13 hours to New York.

I came home, went to London at 17 to work for the summer with my aunt Peggy. She was a manager at the Kingsley Hotel where a lot of high society and film stars stayed. I stayed one week and escaped back home. Being a chambermaid wasn't for me.

At 18 I went on to college to study chiropody in England, and when I graduated, I came back to do my practical training and that's where I met Walter, my future icon. He was a well-travelled man, very eccentric in his mannerisms. He learned all his qualities of healing in Egypt and passed these on to me. However, when I trained with him something was still amiss.

Then I discovered Pauline Willis, a colour therapist from the Hygena School of Colour. I studied with her for 2 years and learned the technique of colour therapy using a reflexology torch on the organs of the body through the workings of the feet. What an amazing therapy which at the time I didn't appreciate fully or realise was my future tool for the success I have had.

When I started my practice, I discovered Jan De Vries, a well-known guru of herbalism. He could diagnose by looking at your eyes. I went to many seminars and did his training in the Vogel range. He once said at a talk he held in the Killyhevlin Hotel in

Enniskillen, 'You don't need me in Fermanagh when you have Christine Allen.' A tribute I thought was not fitting for me.

But recently, this week, I had a client now in her late 30s who said she first saw me when she was 12 years old at the Killyhevlin with her mum that night and she is still attending with her family now.

Then in 1994, New Vistas, now one of the best companies in homoeopathic medicine, started trading in Limerick. And today it is still, in my opinion, the best in homoeopathic medicine.

I have completed courses with them. A company owned by Martin Murray, their service is exceptional. Mostly next-day delivery to most parts of the UK and their expectation is very prompt if diagnosed correctly by a practitioner. Later on, I will give advice about my experiences with the products.

So, after I finished studying, I went to work with Walter Hynes and he taught me all the qualities I have today. Initially I was known as the 'back woman'. I seemed to be able to put in pulled muscles, mainly in the back, neck and knee areas. I continued to do this work for many years. People came from all over to see me. Word of mouth was my advertisement.

Through doing all this work I gradually introduced my earlier therapy which worked wonders. At 21, I married and had two children. I'm now a grandmother with three lovely grandchildren.

My daughter, at the age of 16, had symptoms of early onset diabetes – thankfully which never developed. I put her on cinnamon capsules and GTF glycamine tablets. She went to do pharmacy at Queen's University Belfast, who asked her during the second semester to do a project on diabetes as they were very skeptical on why she never had to go on medication for diabetes. I helped her with it, and today a second year of pharmacy alternative medicine has been introduced.

A hotelier with a sore back

After starting my practice, I did a monthly clinic in Omagh, where I gained a lot of clients who to this day still come to me for treatment. During my work I had two excellent receptionists, Benadette Quigley and Yvonne Johnston. Initially going back to the clientele that I carried out muscle work on, I started to introduce tissue salts for various forms of inflammatory conditions relating to their problems and from there on to dietary issues. One particular case that stands out in my mind is a young hotelier who had a very sore back. He couldn't straighten up, and it was during the week of the Christmas party nights. He called me up and asked if I could see him urgently. I discovered he had a very inflamed lower pelvic muscle. I told him to go home and put a large green cabbage leaf over the area and leave it on for one night and gave him biochemic no 10 homoeopathic tablets to take every 4 hours. I went in to a Christmas party the next evening and there was no back pain when he was turning around. He laughed and told many people about what I had done for him.

Needless to say, he sent me a lot of clients, so many I could not cope with.

From then I decided to introduce the tissue salts, diet and herbal remedies into all aspects of my work. Later in the book, I will give you my questions and answers in a detailed way so that you all can benefit from them yourselves.

So today I am now in a position to help you who cannot avail of my services. This has shortened my working level greatly as I suffered a heart condition 4 years ago which has stalled me from continuing to be of help to my clientele who supported me through tough times.

Flower remedy studies

About five years ago I studied flower remedies with the well-known Clare G Harvey who herself has had a very successful practice working with the great-granddaughter of Dr Bach where she studied the Bach flower remedies and went on to the essences of the bush flowers and then her own compilation of flower essences of Australia. She came many times to my practice to carry out her own clinic.

There are a total of 66 remedies which can be used singly or in a combination depending on the problem one has. One can access these on the website through Clare G Harvey or from New Vistas, Limerick.

This was where I learned how to prepare my own combinations for various emotional conditions. I still do a varied selection of these throughout my day working and testing for homoeopathic remedies with very successful results. I find them in practice very effective for young babies and children as you will discover later in the book from the testimonials.

Having been back and forth to England recently, sitting waiting on my flight, I look around and I can see people all on mobile phones and laptops or with earphones in – so little conversation.

It's no wonder the world is convulsed with stress and lack of conversation.

Where has the friendly smile and that hello gone – how do we ever strike up a friendship with anyone? It's no wonder we all suffer at some point with those symptoms, say SAD (seasonal affective disorder) which leads to loneliness and depression.

Mental alertness

Communication is the key to our mental alertness, not the electromagnetic field around us being condensed down where we issue blame to other things i.e. colleagues, work, family, causing our heads to be fried with what I call 'the tumble dryer' feeling. All other illnesses come from the electromagnetic rays around us.

A remedy I recommend for this is electroguard or algin. Algin is available from New Vistas and is advised to take daily to protect your natural magnetic field around you and allow your natural energy to work better in your body.

Our bodies need good oxygen to be able to fight against the many pathogens attacking us on a daily basis. If we don't do this then our immune systems become less responsible to feed our other required daily functioning organs, adrenals, kidneys, liver, respiratory and especially our lymphatic systems and digestion.

I have had excellent results using these up to the present day. I will speak about many of these later on.

Moving on, now my next approach to helping you all are the many health issues I have been approached with through the past 35 years.

In this section I will give you answers to the many health conditions I have come across and been asked about for alternative advice.

Another supplement I want to add here is 5-HTP. Over the years I have discovered 5-HTP taking it myself from around the age of 35 – I did not experience the awful word 'menopause', this

I put down to having 5-HTP as I regulated my oestrogen levels. And I

didn't experience those dreaded hot flushes that combined with reducing the high starch in my diet especially potatoes, bread, bananas and coffee.

There are 2 types of 5-HTP. One is called Serotone 5HTP. This helps with emotional strains mainly in relation to depression, social behaviour and bipolar.

The one I took was 5-HTP which is only tryptophan. This is a form of amino acid and it works 30 minutes after ingestion, best taken in the morning. However, if one's sleep is broken due to hormone levels, one at bedtime may help also. Best obtained from Nutri Advanced.

Benefits of adrenal liquescence

Another product I took was adrenal liquescence. This I found very beneficial to anyone waking up during the night sweating and exhausted in the dawn of the day wondering how you can do a day's work. Taking 20 drops of adrenal before bedtime will help solve this issue and works for males or females. Available only from New Vistas.

Thyroid liquescence is very beneficial to those who have a borderline underactive gland. It is very beneficial to balance this and also take selenium and a few almond nuts daily. As thyroxine keeps the metabolic weight low and finds it difficult to balance weight even with exercise.

Psychological warfare remedy

The Feet I Have Felt began with the coronavirus crisis and homeopathy. And in all this I found a remedy for hyoscyamus (psychological warfare). The spirit said, 'Don't realise how much knowledge I have accepted over the years to write it down and pass it on.' I have worked as a homeopath for the last 35 years. God is working through me. Constantly people say that I have been given a gift from God. I will continue to do this work. It claims to raise the pH of drinking water by using electrolysis to separate the incoming water from the tap into acid/alkaline components.

Rod Briggs: mind alert

In 2011, I had the great pleasure to be introduced to the late Rod Briggs from South Africa who practised all over the world doing seminars called mind alert. At first I thought this was just gobble-dygook, but sitting in a room with a hundred people I sure was blown away. He had given an introductory talk and the decision was left to oneself whether it was for one or not. Mind alert deals with the subconscious. Where you can sort out your fears, your outcomes and even healing. It's a process involving breathing and the colours of the rainbow.

Find the most peaceful place to be. Start by taking three deep breaths in. And being very relaxed you start visualising the colour red, orange, blue, green, violet and indigo. Then imagine you are going down a set of steps. Count to 21, and you are at your peaceful sense. Here you can get totally relaxed. Then go down another 7 steps and you come to a lift. Step in, have a quick shower and step out into an empty room. This is your workshop. In the right-hand corner is a lift. It opens and out comes a helper. You know this person. Close the lift and reopen it. A second person appears. You may or may not want these people so you can send them back and ask for replacements.

Here you ask these helpers to sort out your difficulties. In front of you on the wall is a screen. Write these problems on the screen. Flick the switch on the side when a white light comes on. Leave this to your helper to sort out. Get back into the lift and go up the 7 steps. Find your comfort place. Up the 21 more steps through the colours and after you take your 3 breaths come back to yourself. This will tell you what and how you feel. It's a program worth trying. It works.

Rod came over here to Northern Ireland at my request and did many seminars over three years helping people in all walks of life. His memories live on now through the Mindlink website.

MY EXPERIENCES: VACCINES / SIDE EFFECTS

Pfizer
Headaches, dizziness (2 weeks)

AstraZeneca
Sickness, tiredness

And again Hyoscyamus alleviates these symptoms. And I find those who take Hyoscyamus since the pandemic seem to have the side effects of having COVID alleviated. So, I advise you to continue it all the time. I have declined taking the vaccine as I take blood thinners and it's recommended to stop them 2 days prior to having the vaccine. Well these recommendations are no longer a risk now according to medical claims. But I declined and continue to take Hyoscyamus and thankfully today I have stayed free from COVID.

Hazel's story
Just after the beginning of lockdown, my best friend Hazel was diagnosed with a tumour in her kidney. I was treating her for

sciatica which wouldn't settle, and I urged her to get a scan privately. And that was the result, got in time. She and I have walked a rocky road for a number of years. And certainly didn't deserve this. Weeks of surgery later, Hazel was doing very well. A very strange year for us all.

Then, in October, Hazel was to start treatment in three months' time. We will have her first scan. On reflection, in 2020 I worked through this awful pandemic and got good feedback from clients. One product I got great results with was Hyoscyamus from contracting the virus and from those who had the virus. One lady came back to me and called it 'the miracle drug'. So yes I'd say it is. My brother and sister-in-law had COVID and again Hyoscyamus did the trick.

And now we have been introduced to the vaccine, which, bear in mind, doesn't cure the virus. It's only to prevent being hospitalised. I personally won't be taking it. I think more research is needed. We are in a new way of life now.

Research in Cork
Then on 26 January I received a telephone call from Martin Murray, director of New Vistas, to inform me that research has been taking place since August 2020 at Cork University and Cork Hospital on cancer patients who have COVID. It found a natural vaccine has alleviated their symptoms. This found that Hyoscyamus and vitamin C are the natural vaccine.

Week beginning 13 April
By now I hope all of us are back to a normal lifestyle as we were invaded by a new virus attacking the whole world, COVID-19.

Being in lockdown for the fourth week, daily I was getting emails, texts and phone calls on what one can take to try and stay as healthy as one can. My theory on this was to keep the immune system healthy no matter how well one feels: ensure that the digestive system is as alkaline as possible, done by drinking 7+ alkaline water.

I discovered 12 years ago a water filter system called Kangen Water. It first originated as PiMag water in small phials you put into your water and take 7 drops daily. This alkalines the entire body. I got great feedback at the time especially from those suffering heartburn.

Then the Kangen Water took over, coming from the same source in Japan. It is not a cure, only an aid to help keep the body's pH level alkaline. My years of experience using this water has helped people with diabetes and stomach problems. And only very recently in the last two years for babies with very bad reflux - make the baby food up with this number 7 water that seemed to alleviate the reflux. I have at the moment one mother who is using this for her 4-month-old son.

Fighting the pathogens

So, drinking alkaline water, in my view, has and will help people who no matter what viruses attack our bodies throughout our lifetimes we have to fight against the pathogens out there to stay as fit and healthy as we can.

KEEPING OUR IMMUNE AND DIGESTIVE SYSTEM WELL

Hyoscyamus, I have tested on many clients and discovered carriers of COVID-19 and others who had its symptoms had led to their immune system weakened with the virus still lingering in the lung or throat. However, it's best to test before prescribing it as every individual is different. Sitting at my table today amidst all this pandemic I do hope in the months and years ahead we never envisage another cycle like this. So I say always keep your body free from disease where possible. We don't want another time like this.

MY MOST IMPORTANT JOURNEY WITH YOU ALL

To share my findings and results with all the clients I've met over the years of my work. These are answers and advice I've constantly come to find and have been asked on a daily basis from babies as young as a month old to the men and women right through every age to their early 90s. People who came every month or every 3 or 6 monthly sessions.

Some listened, some obeyed and some tried to bluff me. But I always caught those out. And as I've been told, 'Don't try, she will always look over those glasses and by god cut you down in two,' and with that humour will say, 'Do you not listen? Do you want to get well or not? Don't come back unless you do what you're told.'

Bearing those comments in mind it's best to listen. So here goes:

Homeopathy and nutrition

Once detoxification is identified, and I do this with my reflexology technique, then I muscle test for the remedy (xenobiotic) best suited to treat the toxic organ and follow up with the liquescence, this will support the function of the undernourished organ and recover more quickly.

Liquescences are low-potency combination remedies derived from multiple sources, specifically healthy organic bovine tissue combined with minerals, vitamins and herbs.

Abscesses

I have only come across 3 types in my career. One, a young teenage boy who had a recurring abscess on the base of his spine. It seemed to reoccur under stress. However, I suggested he took BAC-Forte and Vermex. The BAC-Forte for the infection and the Vermex for any parasites that may be present in the abscess. In around 4-6 weeks it all cleared up. It only reoccurred if he got stressed again. But thankfully today he is clear.

Acne

I had two young teenage boys suffering with acne vulgaris. This is an inflammatory condition of the glands in the skin affecting the face, arm, back, neck and chest. After testing both boys I discovered a low testosterone level and prescribed an alternative hormone therapy that cleared both boys' skin up. Male Liquescence and again BAC-Forte and Vermex.

In young girls I have found that the endocrine system is lacking in minerals and hormonal levels are low. Female liquescence for the endocrine system followed up with vitamin B works very well. Again, diet seems to play a big role. Avoid wheat, crisps, chocolate and pork, but drink plenty of beetroot and carrot juice. Dress salads with olive and rapeseed oil. Use eggs sparingly. Oat and spelt bread is much better for digestion, made with buttermilk. Natural yoghurt, avocado, pears, green veg, peppers, protein, chicken, white fish and turkey. Avoid too much red meat as it takes 10 days to fully digest in the gut.

Anaemia

Anaemia is a condition marked by reduced numbers of red blood cells or of low haemoglobin in the bloodstream which in turn slows the oxygen transporting around the body. The person may feel a lack of energy and listlessness caused by a lack of iron. Pernicious anaemia symptoms could be characterised by lesions on the spinal cord, weakness, diarrhoea, sore tongue and numbness in the limbs. Therefore vitamin B12 is the supplement for this. In addition, supplement the diet 3 times a week with a dessert of four dried pears (sulphur free) soaked in red grape juice. Eat a raw egg beaten with red grape juice 3 times a week.

Also Alfavena tablets, or Ferrum Phos 6x and Kali Phos No 6.

Anxiety issues

In my life's working experiences none better than the flower bush remedies are excellent. I find after listening to people, sometimes I make up a remedy to meet the symptomatic needs the body needs to repair the issues.

RELAXATION AND POSITIVE CHANGE

As I mentioned earlier in *Through the Feet That I Have Felt* calm, relaxation and positive change will help. Here is a list of remedies that may also help for panic, nightmares or psychic attack.

Alpine Mint Bush
Feeling mentally and emotionally exhausted and a lack of joy. I found this along with Banksia Robur excellent for anxiety. Also ANX and AST. All are available from New Vistas. Very successful especially for those feeling weighed down due to burnout.

Autumn Leaves
Using this I found it beneficial to those to hear, see and feel communication from the other side. Helps to let go and move on in a very profound way.

Blackeyed Susan
For those always on the go impatience also balances the adrenal glands.

Boronia

If grieving over broken relationships try this along with Sturt Desert Rose, especially if going through the loss of a loved one.

Crowea

For individuals who constantly worry and are feeling out of balance brings calmness and vitality again.

Dog-rose

Promotes confidence.

Dog-rose of the wild forces

For niggly fears, promotes confidence.

Fringed violet

For shock and trauma.

Grey spider flower drops

Twice daily will give calmness and courage.

Monga Waratah

Brings calmness and inner strength to the inner core.

Mountain Devil

For hatred, jealousy, anger, holding grudges and suspiciousness. This will bring inner forgiveness and contentment.

Red Suva Frangipani

For turmoil in one's self caused by emotional upheaval and sadness.

Southern Cross

For those who think life has been hard on them and feel hard done by.

Sturt Desert Pea

For deep hurt, sadness and emotional pain.

Sturt Desert Rose

The guilt essence, including for sexual guilt.

Sunshine Wattle

For those feeling life is a struggle and feeling trapped in the past.

Tall Mulla-Mulla

Feeling scared, unsafe – this will help to bring the ability to interact with others and feel secure with those people.

Tall Yellow

Top for loneliness and feeling isolated and will bring a sense of belonging.

Turkey Bush

Those who don't believe in themselves and have a creative block – this will give renewed confidence and ability to be yourself.

Wedding Bush

For relationship difficulty whether it is work, social, intimacy – Wedding Bush will help to restore balance.

Wild Potato Bush

The remedy to help those who feel physically weighed down will help to move on. Also this is very good after childbirth for cleaning the pelvic area.

Wisteria

For women who find intimacy difficult. Also for that macho male will help bring gentleness and enjoyment.

Yellow Cowslip Orchid

Helps clear the pituitary area of the head that endures critical, judgemental, bureaucratic attitudes. Will help step back and develop a sense of arbitration.

I use the remedies today especially those experiencing stress problems, bereavement, energy depletion. The following are the most combined formulae which help with the above however, some single remedies are advisable:

Calm and relax

This is very good for broken sleep. Stress from work or family issues. Stress of schoolwork and exams. Facing an interview or performing in public.

Detox

Excellent remedy for when the body has been overdoing it on carbs or caffeine or alcohol. Also very good for lymphatic drainage and when going on long-haul flights.

Dynamic

Excellent for a quick pick-me-up especially after an illness, post-operation or under a lot of stress at work.

Emergency

This has a calming effect on the mind and emotions during a crisis we are faced with. Allows you to cope better. I remember giving this to one man who couldn't cope with losing his daughter to marriage. He took it about two weeks prior to the wedding and on the day. The tears were very little in comparison to what they were months prior to the wedding.

Positivity

Most definitely will help one's low self-esteem and bring out the confidence one seeks, will lift that shyness one has that prevents speaking out and being comfortable around those who tend to push you back.

SUNDAY 20 FEBRUARY 2022

Inspired by Hazel

I sit at my table facing a picture of my best friend Hazel who I talked about at the beginning of lockdown. Well, 18 months on Hazel fought and fought but that gruelling disease finally took her gentle spirit away from us. Three nights after her funeral she appeared to me in a dream. I saw her face smiling down at me holding my A5 writing pad – that was a sign to me to get back to that book I had abandoned when she became ill when treatment failed her. So, my darling dearest best friend Hazel, I'm today starting the end journey for you that we talked about so much. I never thought you'd leave us.

We sat in the summer sunshine looking at the beautiful white butterflies floating around you. You used to say, 'What are they doing?' I thought they were there to keep you well, and they

did until you saw your new grandson come into this world and hold him with your love that you have given to all your grandchildren.

Hazel always smiled through her fears and hopes. Her famous

words were, 'I'll be fine.' Well, Hazel, I know today you are fine and I will be too when I finish this book for you. Everyone knew Hazel from her many years of success running the Jolly Sandwich in Enniskillen. Far and near visited to try her tasty dishes day-in, day-out. She received many food awards over the years prior to COVID. Today it is still just as successful with the running taken on by her daughter Carina and very dedicated staff. If you are reading this page and ever visit Enniskillen, pop in and have a treat and I assure you that you won't be disappointed. Sign her visitors' book.

Devastating news

One year after the death of my good friend Hazel, I myself had been diagnosed with breast cancer. I suddenly felt a small mark on my right breast area just before Christmas. I left it to 9 January when I made an appointment to see my GP and an amazing lady she was, she red-flagged me to the breast clinic in Altnagelvin in Derry/Londonderry where I went through several mammograms and biopsies. That day I knew that it was cancer. I had known from day one of finding it, by this stage one week later the breast was dropped and discoloured.

Mr Diggin, my consultant, told me one week onwards I had a very angry aggressive form of cancer and one week onwards was back and had to have a mastectomy and lymph nodes extraction. He suggested he would take the left breast as well for precaution. This, I wanted from day one myself. Two weeks onwards again I was in for surgery. One week after surgery I am doing great, and I was down from the moment I opened my eyes post-surgery. No pain but had 4 drains in and then one week later were are out. I have been taking INJ for pain and bruising.

Arthritis and inflammatory conditions of the body

There are so many types of arthritic conditions. Many of which I feel start from poor pH levels or genes passed through the blood plasma. Recently, for fibromyalgia I start with stress and try to source out the root cause and treat it. And I have prescribed AST Anti Stress Remedy, connective tissue liquescence, if necessary AIT anti-inflammatory or PFX, natural pain relief for inflammatory arthritis all available from New Vistas.

We have tried so many alternatives. Turmeric will ease inflammation only. Glucosamine will slow down the wearing away of the cushion on the joint. Joint liquescence is very good overall. The homeopathic remedy I have got results with especially for knees and again connective tissue joint and AIT with Amino Acid have proven successful for me.

Bladder and bowel concerns

Bladder issues usually arise when post-menopause is near. Through my reflexology and colour laser therapy, I have had great success with lifting up the bladder wall. A session on a monthly basis certainly proved successful for many of my clients. Sometimes in combination with bladder sarcodes (available from New Vistas). If not on blood thinner or heart medication – dandelion drops are excellent, 15x2 daily. If kidney infections are an issue I suggest

Bac-Forte with kidney liquescence 1x3 (New Vistas). And if it's urinary tract infections Bac.Forte with urinary liquescence.

Men can use these also if experiencing these issues. I also suggest keeping to a fairly alkaline diet. When constipation is a problem, this can be many things: stress, a congested colon, ileocecal valve, liver (fatty), water.

Stress. Again, look at what this is (work, family, hormones). After one addresses the stress, look at the diet: too many carbs i.e. in sugar, bread, potatoes. Too many citrus fruits or additives. So regular colon cleansing and avoiding caffeine as this only enhances the stress and doesn't relieve it as many may think is recommendable. You can use a colon cleanse for up to 2 weeks only and drink plenty of pH water. Not carbonated and also avoiding all of the above. Use colon liquescence from New Vistas or colon capsules from health shops. All these will improve things. I usually recommend magnesium citrate daily and Opsin II and this stops the attack of aggravated food from adhering to the colon wall. Drink up to 1.5l daily.

Green tea

I use green balance tea from the Yogi company. I find it a very cleansing refreshing tea in the morning. If one has been having alcohol the evening before with a meal or have been at a function this will help to clean the liver and digestive system. Also, Hepex is very good for cleaning the liver. It not only is alkaline but breaks up fat of the liver allowing the bowel to work easier.

Jaundice, diabetes, hepatitis, cirrhosis

Another issue that is very common today associated with the bowel is Candida. Again, follow the guidelines on the constipation page and take a good prebiotic that has insulin in it with a prebiotic, dairy-free preferably. I also prescribe Candida drops alongside the above daily until the condition clears.

Cholesterol in the body is essential

But the level must be balanced. If cholesterol is above 6 points, then some attention is needed. It is a much-blamed and misunderstood condition. The loose particles which travel through the artery are dangerous and could possibly cause a stroke. The lining on the inside of the arteries is usually caused by alcohol, nicotine and amino acids, i.e. egg whites, too much red meat.

NEW VISTAS

LIMERICK BASED COMPANY

New Vistas have a supplement of red yeast rice which has proven very effective at reducing cholesterol. It contains brown rice flour with chromium picolinate. This helps the body process carbohydrates and fats resulting in keeping type 2 diabetes and weight loss under control. Also advisable is to take magnesium nitrate which will aid with cramps in the legs and circulation control.

Gout

Another association with fat lipids in the blood known as uric acid, a great old remedy was a glass of raw potato juice in a good AIN anti-inflammatory. First thing every morning and avoid the foods I explained earlier for cholesterol. Also body pH neutralises the other acid in the blood.

Crohn's disease

Another very painful autoimmune disease – bacteria in the digestive tract that causes the body's immune system to attack your healthy cells can occur at any age usually between the ages of 20 and 30 and can also be genetic. Wholegrains and high-fibre foods can cause a traffic congestion in the gastrointestinal tract leaving open pores in the wall. I suggest small and large intestine drops 7x3 daily. Avoid the above foods and sometimes take a digestive enzyme. If one has a lot of diarrhoea or stomach bloating, L-glutamine 500mg, is very helpful. Sometimes a good probiotic is also very good.

Colitis and diverticulitis

Colitis and diverticulitis is chronic inflammation in the sigmoid colon which causes pain and inflammation in the abdomen (stomach) usually in the lower left side flaring up usually a/ 40 and over age bracket b/ obese c/ a chronic smoker who takes little exercise d/ have a diet high in animal products or those on a low fibre diet.

Try to avoid all pork, red meats and dairy. Eat poultry, fish and eggs – best to eat spelt bread or oat bread if you can digest oat. In my experience of treating this condition I have advised to eat the above and use lactose-free, almond or rice milk. Avoid cold salad foods i.e. iceberg lettuce, melon, cucumber. Instead have a warm salad with green beans, tomato, brown rice, beetroot and potato (without the skin).

When the wall of the intestine becomes very porous one will experience gas, bloating, possibly diarrhoea, frequent bowel movements and fatigue. So I advise: small and large intestine 7x3 daily Manuka Honey high strength daily. Yarrow Complex or Opsin I to prevent attacking of food to the intestine.

AIN anti-inflammatory drops if the inflammation is chronic. Also regular reflexology on a 6-week appointment basis is successful, in conjunction with the above.

Blood pressure

There are two types. High blood pressure, firstly, which is the most common. Most high blood pressure comes from stress (work, home, social). In my experience, as I suffer with blood pressure myself as I had a severe blood pressure attack 4 years ago and ended up in hospital with severe angina and thyroid problems – it is quite genetic as it is quite evident in my family. However, I am on 4 BP tablets daily and 2 angina tablets, 1 thyroxine and blood thinner tablet. I do take homoeopathic remedies, the main one for stress AST 3 times daily and Hepex to keep my liver cleansed of the adverse toxins of the drugs. So one can take homoeopathic remedies alongside these meds. However, avoid if on diuretic or blood thinning meds. But always seek advice with the company or practitioner prior to trying these.

Low blood pressure, secondly, is very hard to treat but I found the homeopathic remedy HYT (New Vistas) is excellent for re-balancing low blood pressure. Heart liquescence is excellent for treating general congestion of arteries, muscle and oxygenation to the heart and lung areas. Another heart product called cardiovascular liquescence keeps the heart and circulatory system in good zinc. These nutritionally help with the imbalance and deficiencies of the heart. They are very gentle and safe, especially for genetic heart failure.

Diabetes

Alternative medicine can be useful for diabetes, but this should not be considered to the exclusion of professional medical help. Any diabetic condition should be treated with great care. The suitability of any alternative therapy depends on the condition of the individual diabetic patient and the medication that person requires. However, I have helped a few diabetics with my homoeopathy which has helped manage their insulin dependency. One female client I have has found that digestive enzymes help with controlling her insulin especially after a night out. She also had COVID twice and said it affected her insulin levels quite a bit. Another young 16-year-old girl I treat who is quite athletic takes amino acid liquescence and this seems to balance her levels and her endocrine system. When she is in her menstrual cycle she also takes female liquescence. I have a 30-year-old male who is also insulin dependent and takes adrenal liquescence twice daily and this helps balance.

Hormone problems

Agnus Castus is also very good at balancing oestrogen and progesterone levels; however, do not take it when using contraception. A good remedy for those with infertility.

Reproductive liquescence is very good for women whose fertility is low. However, sometimes it is good to use the uterus formula from New Vistas. I have had good success using these formulae. It is always good to cleanse the uterus wall and fallopian tubes.

Hot flushes

I do find MNO (New Vistas) excellent. HHC is also very good if both levels of oestrogen and progesterone are low. To know which one is most suited, with HHC the symptoms will be tiredness, mood swings, sleep imbalance, stiffness and bone pain. MNO is usually just for the hot sweaty feeling in the body. Dong Quai is for premenopausal women who experience changes in the reproductive system and is also very good for cysts and polycystic ovaries. In China and Japan women use this product from their mid-20s and very seldom experience menopause issues. Female liquescence is another very good formula for young females aged between 16 and 25 who experience PMT irregularities in their cycle. Overall immune system Liquescence is excellent at recovering from the aftereffects of flu.

Immunity

The immune system tells a lot about one's wellbeing. Once I would have said the immune system thrived on good wholesome food i.e. fresh fruit, nuts and vegetables. Especially when we were in the throes of COVID-19 ,it hasn't gone away. And I see every day what this virus has done to the immune system. People cannot fight the common cold, keep getting head colds, sinus and ear problems, sore throats, phlegm on the chest, breathing difficulties, headaches and muscle pain.

My plan I have given with good results are first to test if the spleen is still underactive and treat with the symptoms each client is experiencing and secondly, give VIR or VIR-Forte alongside immune, booster or IMS – these will help to alleviate the symptoms and generally the client will feel more energised and a feeling of wellbeing again. If the glands in the neck, throat or tonsils are giving an issue I recommend treating the thymus gland with Thymus Liquescence and Calendula Complex.

For tiredness and lack of get up and go, feeling sleepy halfway through the day and not sleeping great at night I find Revive Active or Zest Active very beneficial, along with vitamin

B12 1000mcg either in liquid, spray or tablet form. Don't take Vitamin B12 if you already have pernicious anaemia for which vitamin B12 is given in injection form. And avoid spinach, raw foods, barley, grass, dairy, eggs, salmon, chicken, meat. Stress also is a big factor in reducing the immune system, this can bring on other serious illnesses in the body, one being mainly cancers of the kidney, colon and lungs. So addressing the stress is a must here.

My wellbeing ranges from New Vistas provide remedies like relaxation, connection and myself which is a good foot to start with in dealing with the stress accompanied alongside the bush remedies or flower remedies I have mentioned earlier in the book on the section about flower remedies.

In doing this I do think the cancers in our body may be controlled with treatment. Bacteria, in my opinion, attacks the thymus gland which is the immune support activator. In the past I have treated the thymus gland in clients who have had several bacteria-recurrent issues and lyme disease and chronic nasal/throat problems. Address the glandular area concerned; treat or prescribe thymus liquescence with Bac-Forte and a sarcode if necessary; decide if it is lung related, heart and lung sarcode; if it is throat, gargle vitamin C liquescence; if nasal use alongside the above with OPSIN II or SNS formulae; if mucus is present use alongside with above mucus liquescence.

Cellulitis

This is an infection caused by bacteria getting into the deeper layers of the skin if a streak or a bruise, cut, graze, insect bite of the legs become painful, very hot and very red. Sits usually treated with antibiotics I suggest to enhance the immune system take immune liquescence twice daily along with Bac-Forte 3 times daily. If finished antibiotics keep the immune system strengthened to avoid reoccurrence.

My father has been in hospital with this condition for 14 weeks but his issue is high potassium which flares the cellulitis up. So he is given potassium binders daily. High potassium is not a condition that is fully curable. Just follow a low potassium diet (no bananas, potatoes, nuts, melon, orange juice, tomato paste, lentils).

Dairy, wheat, sugar, caffeine, monosodium glutamate in drinks and foods.

I suggest eliminating the above from the diet. First while doing this, I suggest you take OPSIN I which is a supplement for helping to eliminate the cause from the body. If the stomach is cramping, windy or bloated, take digestive enzymes or small and large intestines if the gut is very porous. If diarrhoea is an issue take AHO and a good prebiotic.

I had a farmer who had a lot of headaches and congested nose and recommended Agritech, a powerful sarcode as I thought the problem was in relation to the dust from silage or hay. It alleviated the problem completely. Pollen or hay fever is another big problem. I suggest from October to the end of February to take the supplement Quercetin daily – this is a natural antihistamine which will build up the resistance to the hay fever, general dust or a very dry heated office area. I suggest OPSIN II with Nat-Sulph.

Dry goosebump skin

For very dry goosebump skin include omega-3 oils in the diet. Use olive oil when cooking. Also use a good hyaluronic moisturiser on the skin in your skincare routine daily looking at the emotional aspect. Try AST (New Vistas) and after a liver detox use glutathione complex to regulate energy and cell nutrition if hormones haven't returned to the normal cycle. Try taking liquescence twice daily also.

Fainting spells

For migraines related to PMT: take female liquescence or if experiencing fainting spells take pituitary liquescence. Pituitary liquescence will help balance part of the endocrine symptom. I have seen this in young teenagers going through PMT and early onset menopause.

Lyme disease

I came across this in two clients during COVID. These men had been out in contact with foresty areas and unknowingly got bitten by ticks causing their joints to swell. One was hand related and the other on the legs, so I suggested Vermex and Borrelia Homocord which actually took out the parasites completely.

Autoimmune is now appearing very regularly since COVID. My findings are an increase in lupus, rheumatoid arthritis and Addison's disease, pernicious anaemia and hair loss.

Addison's disease is when your immune system attacks your adrenal glands; if 40% of your adrenal cortex is damaged, your adrenal glands cannot produce enough of the steroid hormone cortisol or aldosterone. Symptoms could be fatigue, abnormal tiredness or drowsiness, muscle weakness, low mood, loss of appetite (weight loss), needing to urinate frequently, increased thirst and craving for salty foods.

Devil's Claw may help alleviate these mild symptoms alongside adrenal liquescence. Do not take Devil's Claw if on heart medication. Pernicious Anaemia is a lack of vitamin B12 in the body. Symptoms may be shortness of breath, rapid heart rate, tingling or numbness of hands or feet, loss of appetite, bleeding gums, impaired sense of smell, unsteadiness when walking and fatigue.

Kidneys

The kidneys require regular cleansing, so drink plenty of alkaline water, Kangen water is excellent. Also use salt sparingly as they burden the kidneys. A strong smell will also indicate too much acid building up in there as a result of too much caffeine, fizzy drinks or eating a lot of carbs. Sometimes it is better to take body pH to alkalise the acid, kidney liquescence to balance the tissue function. If kidney grit or stones present a problem, a supplement KDS is effective. Also drink aloe vera juice and dandelion tea.

Sometimes women can be prone to frequent UTI infections, urinary symptom liquescence twice daily to promote health and vitality again.

Another common problem I recently have come across is where men are experiencing constant urinating at night and their prostate gland is not posing an issue. In this instance I have found kidney liquescence taken twice daily and no caffeine at night a very successful outcome.

Constant sore throats can lead to a weakness in the left kidney.

Using the above remedies will also help with this. Foods to avoid if anyone has any of the above issues with the kidney

are chocolate, tea, tomatoes, spinach, broad beans, asparagus, broccoli, rhubarb and strawberries.

Albumen is a blood protein. If this gets too low fluid is retained and oedema occurs in the feet, ankles and lower legs. So avoid eating the whites of eggs. Glutathione complex is a good tonic for the kidneys.

Liver disorders

The liver is one of the organs I come across in my work – fatty liver and toxic liver.

Fatty liver: A fatty liver has become very common and is not always related to food or alcohol. Non-alcoholic fatty liver usually has no symptoms – patients may complain of tummy pain, pain in the lower back and feeling tired. I usually prescribe Hepex which I have found generally clears this up in about 6-8 weeks and advise to stay on it once a day. Red yeast rice also will help if it is related to high cholesterol, diabetes or high blood pressure.

Toxic liver symptoms are: yellow colour of the skin, itching, loss of appetite, tiredness, a rash, nausea and swelling in the legs or ankles. In this case I usually prescribe a liver cleanse by taking ginger and lemon tea, an oatmeal drink, turmeric drink and green tea.

Lymph system

The lymph glands can swell up during infections and this is always an indication that help is essential. Also during the course of the day, a large amount of toxic material can gather up in the glands. So either take Lympex or Lymph liquescence. Calendula is also very good to take to clear the throat, lymph area or if you are experiencing itching on the palms of the hands or feet. Lympex for overall lymph build-up and maintenance especially if continuous itching occurs in hands or feet.

Lymph liquescence

When a person is sore to touch around the body i.e. fibromyalgia or ME, this remedy is very good to take and reduce the build-up in the muscle tissue. And as you can read about my experience in the next chapter I found the lymph liquescence a wonderful aid in my drainage after surgery.

Male issues

Prostate and low sperm counts. In my findings the prostate can sometimes stem from low kidney and adrenal function due to stress. So, if I am introduced to a male who has a lot of acid secretion I usually suggest to alkalise the kidney, adrenal and prostate before suggesting prostrate formulae. Also take zinc and eat almond and pumpkin seeds daily.

Young men who have fertility issues, also use it for migraine, headaches, ear infections and anxiety.

Yogi Green Balance

Yogi makes a good tea called Green Balance which is an ayurvedic blend of green tea, lemongrass and peppermint and also contains kombucha which is very refreshing on the liver. I take a mug of this every morning. Also very effective if one feels a hangover after a night out. Also milk thistle is also very good – 15 drops twice daily will help over a monthly stint. It also protects the liver.

Recommended foods are: artichokes, potatoes, natural brown rice, honey, berries and black grapes and carrots. Do not use tea, coffee, white sugar, white flour and food made with it, spices, cucumber, cauliflower, cabbage, spinach, pork and chocolate (milk). After 6 weeks try to introduce some of the above back into the diet.

The effects steroids can have on the liver will slow down the metabolic rate. Long-term use may cause non-alcoholic liver. In this case follow the above on fatty liver issues. Kali Mur also can help.

Abdominal migraine

This is a condition common among children who experience constant stomach pain, symptoms, nausea, vomiting, loss of appetite and a pallor to skin colour in young children. It could be anxiety issues e.g. bullying or trauma. New Vistas have recently added a new spectrum of My Wellbeing remedies targeting the mental clarity and emotional distress one envisages on daily perception. In this case of abdominal migraine in children the wellbeing remedy (anxiety) would be beneficial as it will target the mindset from traumatic thoughts to calmer emotions.

Male liquescence

A very good remedy for men who have a low sperm count or low libido. KPA is another good remedy from New Vistas for young males who suffer with acne rosea on the body and cleanses the toxins from the kidney area also while enhancing the male testosterone levels. Also take the zinc citrate and pumpkin seeds two tablespoons daily over the cereal. I find in my daily work with men a lot of them have an over-acid system and this causes low pelvic backache especially for men in the construction business. So I recommend Body pH (New Vistas) 7 drops, 3 times daily for one month only.

The pancreas, I find with many clients, an issue in relation to digestive issues as a lot of people today tend to eat a high-carbo-hydrate diet and this slows down the digestive enzyme or system function which can cause tiredness, headaches, wind and bloating (flatulence) and cravings.

In these cases I suggest taking one digestive enzyme daily and magnesium citrate in the evening. Some non-insulin diabetics find the formula DIN excellent for maintaining the blood sugars alongside pancreas liquescence. Pancreas liquescence is also good to take if you have the threat of being pre-diabetic.

Menopause

Many women experience early menopause or perimenopause from as early as age 37-58, of which I have had many in my clinic. Every woman is different with different symptoms.

One notably can be feeling warm at night with irregular sleep. I sometimes recommend MNO if I think this is the case along with adrenal liquescence or HHC if it's an oestrogen drop in the hormones along with adrenal liquescence. Other women who are still having a cycle can still experience a large dip in energy and mood and loss of libido. Here I would recommend going back to my flower essences or take female liquescence with rhodiola or ashwagandha and kali-phos. And also there is a formula called libido liquescence which works for both males and females.

Women over the age of 60 sometimes have a dip in progesterone levels which again I have had to deal with. In these cases, I prescribe progesterone drops which balance the levels again and allow the bone density levels to remain fairly stable. These drops help keep the bladder wall from prolapsing.

A lot of women still like to take Evening Primrose and Starflower/Borage oil but I don't find these as effective, only my opinion.

Another supplement I recommend at these stages is magnesium citrate to help with the bowel and with sleep. And bone liquescence especially if pineal osteoporosis is an issue. Use Kalisulph for vaginal discharge.

Migraines

A very wide complex health condition. A lot of migraines are caused by allergies i.e. diet, dust, chemical usage.

Pregnancy

I do a lot of reflexology for pregnancy. I only start the regime after 15 weeks and the first scan is done. Reflexology is excellent for pregnancy up until hospital admission. It helps throughout the process of labour. During the trimesters I suggest taking one digestive enzyme daily. Two weeks prior to full-term I suggest Arnica 30 twice daily or INJ this helps with the pain of labour and internal healing afterwards for up to two weeks. In my findings of prescribing the digestive enzyme, babies do not suffer with reflux or wind problems, they are more settled and very contented. During pregnancy if nausea is an issue, then take Nux Vomica

D3 twice daily.

Prostate

Prostate problems are now a very common issue in men. I see daily a lot of men from their mid-50s to their mid-70s with a lot of issues. Unexpected enlarged prostate – some men are born with an enlarged prostate. The prostate is made up of tiny glands as well as muscle and fibrous tissue; the main function of the prostate is to secrete nutritious fluids required for the transportation of healthy semen.

Prostate liquescence: also take 12 citrate daily as it is an excellent homoeopathic remedy designed for the purpose of containing and overcoming prostate irregularities (New Vistas).

It also will help with constant urges to urinate, especially at night. I tell men to avoid drinking too much beer or lager late in the evening, also Coca-Cola or Lucozade.

Prostatitis

This is a condition when an infection occurs and becomes inflamed. I suggest in this case taking Bac-Forte 7 drops 3 times daily and AIN 10 drops twice daily.

Phlebitis/cellulitis

A condition caused when inflammation of a vein, or veins, occurs can be very painful. AIN (New Vistas) is very good to take alongside AIT if the area is itchy. Use Vermex to erase the parasites (which can cause the itchiness) if it is related to a build-up of toxins in the blood use Sanguinex to clean the blood. Tiredness and restlessness also can contribute to vascular issues. Take Vitamin E

400-500 IB and also 5mg of folic acid (twice daily both). If legs are twitching, magnesium phosphate 6x will help keep the blood alkalined. Also, if the symptoms still persist, introduce Calc Phos 6x and this will help greatly.

Polycystic ovary

Polycystic ovary syndrome usually occurs in women aged between their early teens and their mid-to-late 20s. Symptoms can be irregular cycle or an absent cycle, irregular ovulation or none, pelvic area weight gain, facial hair, oily skin or severe acne and thinning of scalp hair.

Women who have these are at a risk of developing type 2 diabetes, depression, high blood pressure and high cholesterol and sleep apnoea. What I usually recommend is female liquescence and KOA. Female liquescence (1 tbsp twice daily) KOA 7 drops 3 times daily.

In cases where facial hair is an issue, I prescribe prostate liquescence once a day. This will reduce the facial hair. Women prone to only ovarian cysts use KOA 3 times daily.

Endometriosis is a painful disorder in which tissue grows outside of the uterus, this tissue thickens then breaks down and bleeds with each cycle. It then gets trapped and this causes the surrounding tissue to become irritated thus developing scar tissue.

Endometriosis is found in the ovaries, fallopian tubes, outer surface of the uterus and bowels and on each cycle can cause severe pain in the lower pelvic region. Reduce the stress in the body. Reduce intake of caffeine and if a smoker try to stop. Note that a high-carb diet is also a risk factor. Do a detox diet, the flower remedies on the detox would be of help. Improve the lymph system, take lymph liquescence twice daily. Balance the pituitary levels by taking either 5-HTP or pituitary liquescence (take 15 drops twice daily) also take balance hormone levels Fempro (New Vistas) or HCG to help natural metabolic response and correct hormone levels.

Stomach disorders

When I first started my practice 33 years ago, homoeopathic medicine was not as advanced as it is today. My first experience was with a client who had a stiff back. Working on him, I asked what he ate. He was a construction worker, laughed and said he came 'with a sore back, not a stomach problem'. I laughed and told him it's related, and at that point I think he thought I was nuts. But to his surprise I told him to stop drinking tea and eating ham, bread and chocolate.

'I'll die of starvation,' he said. 'Not a bit of you. Do you want to get better? Then do as I say.'

And I put him on biochemic tissue salts no 10.

After a week he called me. His back pain was gone, and I saw him quite recently and he said: 'I'm still off the tea and ham.'

A lot of stomach issues are diet related and in turn damage the digestible enzymes needed to help break down food into smaller molecules so that they can be absorbed into the body. These are made by the pancreas.

I find a lot of pancreatic insufficiency to digest their food hence leaving issues with headaches, tiredness, bloating and unable to break down starch in the diet.

Address this by:

- Cutting down on high-starch foods i.e. bread, pasta, rice, dairy chocolate, chips, potato.
- Drinking water, decaffeinated drinks.
- Opting for wheat-free pasta and breads.
- Eating papaya fruit daily.
- Taking a digestive enzyme daily.

I usually recommend either marshmallow and Gamma Oryzanol or Simalese from Nutri advanced or Digestive Enzyme liquescence from New Vistas.

Sinus and lymph system

Now this is a complicated one. Sinus can come from diet, stress, pollution, asthma-related issues. All of which I've come across over the years and sometimes from gum issues which I recently discovered. A good reflexologist can tell you which of the above it could be. So testing after lymph drainage is the best tool to find out which it is. If it's diet, illustrate a daily wheat-free diet and dairy-free and food additives (have a lot of sugar)

Fructose, dextrose, lactose, maltose, sucrose, galactose

If it's stress, address it with tryphon 5-HTP Seratone supplement (also hay fever from New Vistas) along with the guidelines works very well. Have reflexology which really helps but also it's important to find out what the main source is. Supplement the diet if needed. SNS and Opsin I are excellent if it's air pollen or dust pollen.

Hay fever and immune booster

From September to March, it is suggested to use quercetin to build up the material antihistamine in the body this will prevent the hay fever from reoccurring to a heightened level.

During the hay fever season if one's eyes swell up and close try Nat Sulph 6x4 drops 3 times daily alongside the hay fever drops (New Vistas) 7 drops, 3 times daily.

Sciatica

Today sciatica is very quickly diagnosed to patients who complain of nerve pain down the leg. In my early days of working with people with sciatica, they could barely walk or get out of bed as the sciatic nerve was compressed by a disc where it had become prolapsed and inflamed causing a protrusion on the nerve root. Anti-inflammatory remedies alongside acupuncture or laser treatment can react well so ANTI with INJ can help.

Shingles

This is something that has become very common since COVID came. I believe it is another viral strain of COVID. Some experience a rash anywhere on the body, others just pain. I recommend VIR FORTE 7 drops 3 times daily along with AST to destress the body and rub the skin with a leek that has been opened. Only use this if the skin is blistered. Eat plenty of leeks also and if this does not clear try Vermex to kill the parasite associated with the virus.

Skin disorders

Usually associated with unanswerable itchy skin anywhere over the body. First thing to do is do a liver cleanse, go back to where I spoke about detoxing the liver. After a liver cleanse if there is persistent itching then look at the stress levels in one's life. Sometimes one has to address the emotional aspect also. I think touch for kinesiology is very good to detect exactly where the locked stress may have occurred that one is not aware of happening during their lifespan. Acne associated with skin is also a very traumatising experience especially in young teenage years. In my experience again, diet, hormone imbalance is usually the key factor. Go back to my area on acne I wrote earlier for both male and female.

Varicose veins

Varicose veins are swollen and enlarged veins that usually occur on the legs and feet. They may be blue or purple and lumpy, bulging or twisted in appearance. Other symptoms include: aching heavy and uncomfortable legs, swollen feet and ankles, burning and throbbing in your legs, muscle cramp in the legs particularly at night and itchy and thin skin over the affected vein. The symptoms can be worse during the warm weather if you are standing up for a long time. What causes the varicose vein to develop is when the small valves inside the veins stop working properly. Certain things can increase your chances of developing varicose veins such as being a female, genetic, being overweight, standing a long time especially on tiled surfaces and can be common in pregnancy.

Vasculaforce by Vogel can help, circulation liquescence by NV twice daily alongside AIT if you have an itch or AIN if inflammation is present. Also keep legs elevated when sitting in the evening. Avoid alcohol, nicotine, spices and salt.

Side effects of medications

These are remedies I have used over the years and found great results with Chemex for reducing the side effects of medications e.g. antibiotics, antidepressants, anti-inflammatory or steroids.

ADI

Excellent for constant diarrhoea.

Agritex

I also had success with this with a client with a constant dry cough, and after taking Agritex 3 times daily after a month the cough cleared. He was a farmer around cattle and hens all the time.

AIN

For inflammation anywhere in the body.

AIT

For constant itch anywhere in the body.

ASM

To help stop smoking.

AST

One of my remedies I recommend daily to clients which is excellent in very stressful conditions e.g. personal stress (family related issues) or studying.

Algin

Excellent remedy for those that have too much electrical radiation around them e.g. mobile phone, laptops, hairdressers.

Chlorex

I recently found this remedy very useful to a client who swam every morning in the local leisure centre and was constantly sinus blocked and had head fog. After using it 7 times a day the head and sinus completely cleared.

EBV

This remedy will detox the Epstein Barr virus-related conditions. Again in my years of work I have found this an excellent remedy for clients who had glandular fever and are still suffering the side effects from it.

Hay fever

Excellent to take at the early onset season of hay fever beginning with Opsin II also.

HC2

Excellent for constipation.

Hemo

For excessive iron levels in the blood, I recently recommended this to a client with great results lessened her having to have too much time taking off each month.

Hepex

Excellent detox for the liver especially when the liver readings exceed the regulated level. I recently recommended this to my brother who had great success with it. Also very good if the liver is fatty.

Opsin I
Very useful to take when detoxing from certain foods in the diet helps to alleviate the attack of food adhering to the gut wall.

Phosphatex
Very good if one is overloaded with artificial sweeteners or those who constantly eat rubbish foods i.e. crisps, fizzy drinks, sweets etc.

Sanguinex
Good for taking toxins out of the blood or doing a blood cleanse.

Body pH
I have recommended this to clients who I find their kidney are very acidic or in one case to a diabetic to help balance his pH level from over slightly acid to alkaline. This helped to keep his blood sugar under control.

Candida
Taken with Vermex or Vermex-Forte for several clients. Candida is excellent.

DIN
Again I have excellent feedback with DIN in supporting blood sugar readings.

HEM
For haemorrhoids.

HHC
Very good for balancing oestrogen/progesterone levels. If one experiences hot flushes it can be very effective.

INJ
Helps to rebuild cellular tissue after surgery. I have experienced this remedy quite recently. After having my mastectomy, I took it every few hours and I had no bruising and my wound healed up in about 2-3 weeks.

IRR
The remedy I have used on a client who is still taking it and it keeps her pulse under 85 where it was previously over 95.

Lupus
Lupus is an autoimmune disease in which the immune symptom begins to ecognize and attack the body's own tissues. No two people can have the same symptoms. Lupus can attack the body from as early as the mid-teens to the 30s and may be mild, severe, sporadic or continual.

Common symptoms include fatigue, fever, hair loss, skin rashes, joint pain, kidney problems and digestive problems.

An antibody test called ANA can reveal if it is positive.

During my years of work I had a colleague who has lupus. She kept a very healthy diet, avoided the strong ultraviolet light in the summertime and took supplements.

Koa

When there is a presence of a cyst on the ovary sometimes this causes the kidney not to flush out properly and then this causes the adrenal gland to get sluggish causing discomfort. Down on the right or left side of the abdomen taking KOA on a regular scale can help with this condition.

KPA

I have prescribed this to a young man in his mid-50s to early 60s who had a kidney removed and who suffered with tiredness and higher readings of PSA. The KPA seemed to reduce the PSA and also lifted the energy levels and release the tiredness.

MNO

An excellent remedy for menopause symptoms especially if experiencing hot flushes and mood swings. Take with AST if you have stressful issues with it also.

PFX

An excellent alternative for pain relief.

SCI

Very effective for sciatica pain – do the leverage exercises alongside taking it, lift up the leg breathe out and breathe in as you lower. Do on both legs separately and then both together.

VTG

Excellent remedy for vertigo or dizziness.

Helicobacter pylori

This remedy is very effective for stomach bugs. Related to helicobacter, needs to be taken for about 2 months for effectiveness.

Borrelia Burgdorferi

A great detox for bites in relation to garden bugs where swelling occurs on the skin; one bottle will usually clear the condition.

Rhus Tox

For inflammation around the joints if a diagnosis of arthritis is not given.

Ruta grava

For mild fractures, breaks or cracks in the rib areas, foot, hand.

Thuja 12x

Very good for warts and verucas.

Kiddies range

Homeopathy is particularly suited and very effective to children for all ages from shortly after birth.

From a few weeks after birth the immune system can be developed and help with the overall growth of the child. They can be applied by a drop under the tongue or directly on the navel. 1-2 drops for babies. 4-6 drops twice daily for children.

These are the remedies I found excellent results with. Colic baby, constipation relief, calm child, breath ease, bacterial infection, baby thrush, food allergies (mainly milk, lactose, wheat), teething time and sleep ease.

I recommend an immune booster to all children who attend nursery through to the end of primary education. Even my own grandchildren have benefited from this remedy.

Injuries and little traumas are excellent for the tumbles and falls little kiddies endure daily should bruising and fear follow.

I'm going to mention Immiflex for children, an excellent supplement for children under the age of 12 as a lot of children complain of constant tummy pains and constant colds or runny noses.

Supplements from the health shop Nature's Choice, Enniskillen, a very well-run health shop owned by Nuala Lilley and her trained staff always on hand to help with the public coming in for advice on their health. I worked above the shop for a few years prior to my heart condition and found it exceptional for clients to be able to go downstairs and avail themselves of the products they may have needed.

The following products are the ones that I found I used on a daily basis with clients:

Nutri Advanced Adreset
To treat adrenal function.

Ashwagandha
Anti-stress tablet. Very good if stress is related to hormone imbalance. It is also in Perimeno Plus.

Berberine 250
May support glucose levels. Also has milk thistle and silymarin in it to help support a healthy microbial balance in the digestive

tract.

BioCare Magnesium taurate 140

Good for mental health. And magnesium malate is excellent for muscular discomfort. It contains malic acid which might lessen muscle pain in people with fibromyalgia.

Candex

Maintains the balance of micro of the intestinal tract especially if prone to yeast problems. If on high blood pressure medication consult with your practitioner.

LAMBERTS

L-Lysine
1000 mg for cold sores one daily.

Bromelian
For help for a dry mouth in relation to poor saliva juices or have bad breath.

Cinnamon
250 1 daily for help with blood sugar levels.

Quercetin
500mg daily. More effective when taken from mid-October to the middle and end of February – acts as a natural antihistamine for the prevention of an onset of hay fever.

GTF 200 µg. Take for the early onset of diabetes. Also very effective with one cinnamon tablet daily.

Zinc plus lozenges
Great for children to keep their immune system healthy.

Eye wise

To maintain normal vision or failing eyesight keeps the protein the macula.

Premtesse

Supplement for women who still have a cycle and experience discomfort pain to the start of the cycle or mid cycle.

VOGEL

Avena Sativa

Another calming effect on the system. Good for those with sleep problems.

Bronchosan

For constant coughing with phlegm.

Centaurium

For stomach acid reflux – good to use with Mastika gum or on its own.

Dandelion

A blood cleanser that is also excellent for bladder prolapse.

Devil's claw

For mild arthritis in the joints.

Dormeasan

Helps with irregular sleep patterns.

Echinaforce
A natural antibiotic.

Hawthorn complex
For controlling blood pressure, a general tonic for the heart. Do not use if on blood thinners.

Hyperiforce/hypericum
Used as a sedative and for mild depression.

Ivy and thyme
For bronchial tubes and mild, recurrent coughing spasms.

Luffa complex
Hay fever symptoms.

Menosan
For menopause symptoms relating to hot flushes and mood cycles.

Milk thistle
A cleaner for the liver. Use 2-3 times yearly.

Passiflora
For those who get nervous prior to exams, interviews or can't relax late in the evening.

Plantago
For catarrh or for ear wax. Also helps for slight damp cotton wool ear sanitation use.

Salidago
Cleanser for the tissues of the kidneys and for mild kidney sanitation.

Spilanthes
For fungus.

Tormentil
Ease stomach cramps and also diarrhoea.

UVA-URSI
For bladder irritation.

Venaforte
For toning the veins in the legs also good for mild phlebitis.

Yarrow complex
This stops food that can disagree with the digestive system

Menohop
Used for women – is good for balancing phytoestrogen this is when flushes are prevalent, for bone pain and sometimes blood lipid levels.

Multi-essentials for pregnancy in women
Ultra probioplex powder is excellent for children with low immunity who are constantly having bugs.

Saccharomyces

Excellent after a lot of usage of antibiotics or anti-inflammatories for the gut or who have an irregular diet.

Theanine and lemon balm

For a calm and relaxing night's sleep.

Veridian

Vitamin B5 200mg anti-stress vitamin good for people on a daily basis who cannot cope with stressful situations in the workplace.

Bladder

Excellent for prolapse bladder constant leaking.

Eyes

For any problems relating to vision, it is very effective. I myself used this when I had very dry agitation on my eyes after my heart issue.

Heart/lung

For those who experienced tightness and lack of oxygen especially after they have had a lung or chest infection.

Orchid (testes)

Effective if a lump is present on either of the testes.

Uterus

I recommend after childbirth or continued heavy periods or miscarriage.

Christine Allen

Muscle ligament, cartilage
Useful when pulled, strained ligament or cartilage after injury.

MIGRANES

There are so many types of migranes up to thirty six different types. The most common migranes are caused by allergies, cervical disalignments, gall bladder and liver problems or mal function of digestive or hormonal problems.

In the first instance it is best to fint the root cause.

Here are some of my findings, make sure your liver is healthy, this can be done by cleansing it once a month. Hepex new vistas is very good for your liver function, liver Liav essence for both liver and bladder.

Hormonal issues,

Dona Quai alongside, vitamins B supplements and liver cleanse. it is also best to avoid caffeine, starch, chocolate, cheese , wine and citrus fruit.
You could take PFX for the pain.

Head migraine (frontal)

PFX along side Pitutary Liqvessence and adrenal Liqvessence is very effective, accupunturenis also an effective relief from these types of migraines,

Sinus migrane

TNY, hayfever from (nv) with sinus, remedy. If dust allergies are present Opsin. it is also reccomended to get an alergyn test done to reduce impacts of headaches.

LIQUESCENCES

Rebuild and strengthen the organ. These are the common ones I daily found excellent results from:

Adrenal liquescence
Which I have mentioned throughout *The Feet I Have Felt* for various low energy levels.

Bone liquescence
For and to aid bone repair and lessen osteoporosis.

Breast health liquescence
For women of all ages who may have heavy thickening of the breast tissue. I recommend this to women aged 35 plus to help keep breast health.

Circulation liquescence
For various conditions DVT, vasculitis, phlebitis or poor lymph drainage.

Cognitive liquescence

Helps to slow down memory loss.

Connective tissue liquescence

I gained good results with this for fibromyalgia, with other supplements.

Digestive enzyme liquescence

Very effective for those who have poor digestion due to eating too much carbohydrates in the diet.

Heart liquescence

If one feels tired, short of breath, no energy and have had your heart checked with the cardiologist and all clear.

Joint liquescence

Very effective when the start of bone wear is present.

Kidney liquescence

Where recurrent kidney infections are common also. Dandelion is good to take also for cleansing of the kidney.

Microflora liquescence

For gut health where one is always feeling bloated and especially if one has helicobacter pylori.

Pancreas liquescence

A good support where one is told of early onset diabetes and on a diet control.

Pituitary liquescence

This remedy I have used on mainly women who have experienced fainting spells around menstrual cycle times or experienced headaches at cycle times also.

Cardiovascular liquescence

I have clients who use this remedy when they have had heart problems in relation to high blood pressure, post heart surgery but must always consult with a qualified practitioner prior to taking this. It helps to keep preventing build-up of plaque of the arteries.

Lymphatic system liquescence

Where the tissue on the body feels tender to the touch, achy and tired.

BIOCARE PRODUCTS

Adreno complex
For adrenal function.

Astragalus
Colds in the upper respiratory area.

Goldenseal Root
For upset tummies good to use if one has helicobacter with a pro-
biotic mentioned earlier in
  Through the Feet I Feel.

Nature's answer
Cat's claw 1-2 ml daily in water for keeping white blood cell count
up. Also for autoimmune conditions. These are the very latest
products proving even by myself as healing with symptoms of
chemotherapy, symptoms of radiotherapy, diabetes, chloresterol
and pain.

Rhodiola Root
Excellent for stress in relation to everyday issues.

MUSHROOMS 4 LIFE

Chaga

Post-radiotherapy acts as an antioxidant.

Cordyceps

For all aspects of the respiratory area.

Maitake

For ongoing chemotherapy treatment.

Shitake

For tumours in the body. Also for Candida, cholesterol, polycystic ovaries. Also good to take post-chemo along with or on its own myco-qi.

Reishi

Sedative pain and inflammation and autoimmune disease for lupus, MS, reactive arthritis, Sjögren's syndrome, type 1 diabetes (acts as an antihistamine) prickly heat.

HEEL PRODUCTS

The few Heel products – a german product line had good success with over the years.

Nervoheel
Nervousness, irritability, PMS and mild menopause, 1x3 times daily only for over 12s.

Oculoheel
Dry eyes, watery eyes, conjunctivitis.

Traumeel
For pain inflammation it is becoming an option for nonsteroidal and inflammatory use.

Vertigoheel
Excellent for vertigo, dizziness, lack of concentration for over the age of 12, take 1 tablet in the mouth every hour not more than 12 times daily. Usual dosage is 1 tablet 3 times daily.

Viburcol

A calming sedative for young children when teething or suffering poor sleep and agitation. Can be used from the age of 1-5 years old.

Chemex forte

To help expel the anaesthetic from my body.

Lymph Liquescence

To help and enhance with drainage.

Recovery Liquescence

To help with the whole readjusting of the body back to normal status.

Bac-forte

To keep infection down. I know these have helped with my recovery and I will continue on Bac for a few months.

My chemotherapy begins

I started chemotherapy on the 23 March. Now I will start bioplasma which is a compound of tissue salts that my body will need to support my body function to restore my health. Also amino acids help to combat the side effects and helps to prevent cell damage.

CASE STUDY

Female hormone

I'm a 14-year-old schoolgirl. My cycle has not started; what would you prescribe?

Firstly, I will do reflexology to see if the endocrine cycle is working, test the ovary cycle and uterus area also the pituitary levels and adrenal function from here. I balance with my reflexology touch and then with my homeopathic skills I'll test to see what is best to take usually. I would have to prescribe reproductive female liquescence with either pituitary or adrenal liquescence if she is very tired or experiencing headaches or itchy skin, pituitary if has had fainting spells.

Another issue I was approached with was a lovely lady in her mid-50s having repetitive cysts on the breast having gone through many tests, but nothing seemed to work. I tested her after doing a session of reflexology and discovered an imbalance on her pituitary gland. I recommend pituitary liquescence twice daily and now after some months she is clear with no symptoms returning.

Those many questions on hot flushes and tiredness – again, not everyone needs the same remedy in most women. It projects with low oestrogen in the hormone system. I recommend ease of starch and wheat in the diet, coffee and red wine which are big contributing factors and stress.

If stress-related I recommend 5-HTP, not the Seratone, just 5-HTP. Serotone 5-HTP is usually in relation to muscle aches and menstrual cramps. Women who have had COVID experienced mucus in their chest. If this mucus dries up it can cause breast cancer so hyoscyamus Viz VC and breast health was recommended. PSA leading in men can occur after having COVID. Lung cancer also another knock-on effect from COVID so again Hyoscyamus viz vic and respiratory liquescence can help avail of this happening. So it is very important to take the natural vaccine. One can view this survey on https://www.ucc.ie/en/oncamie/.

My Wellbeing are products I recently introduced to my practice with great success.

They combine wellbeing nutrition alongside my other homeopathic remedies, herbal medicine and reflexology and promote emotional and energetic composure and personal stability to one's daily routine of stresses we encounter.

The following are the combinations I have had great success with, with some of my clients.

Myself

Clarity of mind is very important. It is the lack of adequate levels of clarity which can lead to distractions such as alcohol or food abuse, bad company, gambling, medication dependence, illegal drugs and unhealthy sexual engagement. These can be the start of our downfall, leaving one feeling alone, sad, lacking in confidence blaming oneself, socially withdrawal – it goes on.

So what we need is a state of mind of calmness and happiness to regain what we want to achieve our ambitions and goals again, in other words getting back to being grounded.

We need contentment to avoid anger, hate and fear to give us joy and happiness to be able to meet with the highs and lows that life throws at us. When we have that we will be able to see again more clearly the joy in living again.

The self will open to protection, have more faith, courage and commitment to challenges we will face. This is where I found myself a fantastic line to getting there and have used on a few clients who were willing to try it. One said in one day she got results.

Anxiety

Anxiety has affected after the pandemic. It has always been there for decades through peer pressure of society where one household has to keep an image for their neighbours, siblings and friends.

Breakdown in homes due to financial problems, repossession, etc. all this causes the mind to worry more intensely.

Stress from the adrenal glands can cause a breakdown in the cortisol levels of the immune system. This can come about from insomnia or excess insulin and cortisol when released together. High blood pressure is a result of breathlessness, fear, fatigue, headaches, mild chest pain, digestive problems in some cases causing Addison's or Cushing disease.

In my findings for anxiety levels all of the above were experienced. So alongside anxiety, wellbeing sometimes needs testing. The adrenals also can be an added remedy or pituitary both from New Vistas. Again, after a day one week I had great success with feedback from 2 clients especially where they had excellent results for mind stability, inner strength and contentment,

Kiddies range

This is a range of products over my years I continually prescribe to my clients' children when issues arose for them.

Colic baby.

1. Constipation relief.

2. Food Allergies.

3. Calm child sleepease

Especially when young children are having sleeping problems and when they go to nursery, preschool, primary – take both together.

4. Chesty baby

Excellent for mucous in the chest, sinuses and digestive tract.

5. Breathe ease

Good to combine with food allergies if it's a food intolerance.

6. Baby thrush

Again this can be related to bacterial oral infection in the mouth.

Cradle cap

Coconut oil every day on the scalp and spray colloidal silver also at teething time. Some babies do get quite a lot of pain when cutting their teeth.

It's always good to have the following remedies in the cupboard for small children.

a. Injuries, to reduce bruising following a fall or tumble.

b. Little traumas.

c. Viral illness to keep for recurring colds, chests, discomfort coughs.

d. Bacterial infection for any infections, minor or major.

e. Immune booster give daily to prevent picking up all the germs around.

All these are New Vistas products dosage for children are 4-6 drops twice daily. 1-2 drops twice daily for babies. All these give prescribed and achieve results with my clients as you can read in the testimonial section.

Mindfulness

I have related this wellbeing remedy to children and young teenagers who have experienced broken home life where they felt they have grown up with memories of blame, shame, low self-esteem, anger and hatred. All this takes over the emotions and stays in the subconscious for years and all this leads to trauma in the mind and takes over everyday living for years ahead.

I have had personal experience of this and today it has been sorted thankfully.

So, compassion and love are essential and required to set release of this imprisonment of the traumatic mind and with mindfulness this can help release the toxic mindset to a more positive experience which they can turn to accept.

Relaxation

In today's rat race of life, people find it hard to switch off. Sometimes a short walk, a short 40 winks, a quick neck massage or even spending time with your dog or cat, with a cup of tea, watching your favourite film or TV soap helps.

Relaxation is also very important for relationships if there is no communication, love and trust breakdown.

There are many supplements on the market to take but Well-being Relaxation allows peace and tranquility, sweeping away fear or worry or stress and allows a deep sense of calm and peace within oneself to be able to dream less and get more relaxed sleep having a refreshed mind and body.

Serenity

Serene people are those who feel grounded and nothing seems to faze them. It's a gift in its own right. They can deal, listen and accept others' reactions.

Acceptance allows tolerance for one to be able to hear and listen to others' opinions, beliefs and even faiths.

I have had clients who hold these attributes and don't realise they affect them in their own daily regime.

When I tested for serenity and gave them a bottle to try it seemed to naturally turn their mindset to a more calm, positive and overall a better control of their ability to share and be more visual to deal with their issues whether they drink or smoke excessively.

Crystals

After my training in reflexology, I studied a course on crystal therapy. Crystals are natural elements that come from the earth. Homemade crystals don't have the earth's energy.

However, they do still have the crystalline structures that retain energy and once you handle the stone all crystal energy will feel to you is all that you need.

There are many colours of crystals and one may be attracted to you, if you find this to be the case it is the one for you.

So, my work with crystals included the rose quartz, the clear quartz crystal, the amber crystal and the amethyst crystal.

I have an amethyst crystal attached to my deceased mother's gold chain which I use for dowsing if I'm unsure as to what my client needs when I'm prescribing homoeopathic medicine.

The rose quartz I have given to many people over the years when they were depressed, could not sleep at night or were very nervous during exams or going for interviews. Also it is very good for encouraging love and deeper friendship into a relationship.

In all cases it always seems to ignite the request or emotional feeling. It can be worn also as a necklace, bracelet or ring.

Clear quartz works with every type of energy. Great to use if meditating, especially in a grid it can be used to cleanse other crystals. It helps with clarifying thoughts and beliefs and improving concentration. On one of the days I was feeling very unwell going through my chemotherapy my friend Megan called in to see me and the first thing she gave me was a clear quartz crystal. I held it for a couple of hours in my hand. I could feel my body sinking into a very good emotional place.

The amber crystal or citrine helps with pain and inflammation, worn as a ring or amber bracelet for this reason. The citrine is one I have in my home standing forward and facing in to encourage prosperity. If you have a business, place it in the cash register to promote propensity for your business.

The amethyst crystal I have found this great for placing on the forehead for headaches, eye problems, stress, insomnia, nightmares. Place under your pillow or again wear around your neck while sleeping.

I have a large amethyst on my hall table to keep negativity out of my house.

There are many other crystals to use and improve your life. The book *Crystals for Beginners* by Karen Frazier is a good place to start.

TESTIMONIALS

Byronica O'Rouke

She's like an MRI machine. She can unearth anything and everything when she is at your feet. I had a condition of severe tiredness. Nothing seemed to help but Christine discovered it was an oil leak at home. She put me on products from New Vistas and I am perfect now.

Pat Crudden

Christine discovered I had a clot in my leg and sent me straight home to the doctor. I spent 9 days in hospital. And I'm still attending her clinic all these years later and she has put me on several homoeopathic remedies for different ailments that have cropped up with success.

Thelma

My family have been going to Christine for nearly 20 years. She has picked up on so many issues the doctors missed. I can't recommend her enough and look forward to reading this book. My grandson needed glasses and didn't realise. Christine picked up on a blockage in the carotid artery and helped with my dad's condition and still on all the New Vistas remedies.

Jill from Sweden

Christine Allen is a fountain of knowledge, an expert in her field and has the biggest of hearts and the one who revealed I was expecting my first child! Her professional advice and homeopathic recommendations have rescued me on many occasions. This book is one you are going to read and re-read. I'll be taking it with me everywhere.

Laura C

Christine is a knowledgeable experienced practitioner whom I have been attending for 30 years. Her diagnostic skills using reflexology and ability to prescribe the appropriate treatment has helped my family's health on numerous occasions. I highly recommend Christine and have 100% faith in her as a reflexologist. She is a kind, caring, empathetic person who has made a difference to many people.

Karen Keys and family

Christine Allen is an amazing woman. I have known her for over 30 years when she came to my aid as a child. Even before I ring the doctors I just have to ring Christine and she knows the problem and is able to recommend something that will help so much. She has been brilliant these past 8 years while I have had my 3 children. All 3 of them had allergies and gut problems and with her guidance and help they have come through it all. Her homoeopathic remedies are second to none, her knowledge of them is fantastic. My husband would have been a bit of a sceptic but now he has great belief in Christine.

Christine Allen is a great friend and is always willing to help anyone with her amazing remedies. It is a privilege to have her as my friend for many years and avail her guidance and therapies.

Why I first started out on my journey and up to 5 years ago I employed 2 very capable receptionists who both had a knowledge in alternative therapies.

Berni was with me for 15 years and she did reflexology and aromatherapy. I attended her frequently myself and between us both were able to keep our wellbeing under control. Then Yvonne came along after Berni. She is excellent in remedial massage and clay treatments. The clay treatments were intense, lasting 2 hours from massage to applying the clay and then finishing off with either the slimming cream or firming cream. All these came from New Vistas in Limerick. They still do the products. I did use the slimming cream and found it very effective for cleansing the intestinal area. Yvonne also did reflexology. Both her and Berni did the colour reflexology which today I think is a big gap where reflexology treatments go.

Jennifer G

I had been attending Christine on a regular basis and the COVID-19 pandemic hit, being a nurse in a busy nursing home I tested positive for COVID before vaccines were rolled out. I had a rough time with it but didn't need hospitalisation and then got my first dose of vaccine and had a severe reaction to it and subsequently ended up with long COVID. Only for Christine's amazing care and expertise alongside New Vistas' homeopathic remedies I don't know where I would be today. She is a remarkable woman in her field.

Dympna M

I first came to Christine 37 years ago and was treated for very bad depression and lack of confidence after a bad car accident. I first started going for weekly treatments and took avena sativa and hypericum from Bioforce. The sessions then went to fortnightly after 4 months which is up to now to keep it under control. Apart from the reflexology treatments, over the weeks and months ahead I continued on the hypericum and avena sativa and I now take kidney liquescence to prevent reoccurring infections I am prone to and COQ10 for brain function.

Zelda

I have been going to Christine Allen for about 14 years, at least 3 or 4 times a year. Christine is great in diagnosing any issues I would have had and giving me remedies to overcome and help with these issues. She was great during my pregnancies, keeping me relaxed and making sure they went smoothly and again giving me remedies for aftercare too. When I was having difficulties in conceiving, she made up remedies which helped for my second son. She continues to make up remedies and advise drops which have helped me emotionally and mentally. She also makes up remedies for my son who was diagnosed with autism 3 years ago. These help with his concentration and control his emotions. He passed the transfer test and is the top of his class of secondary school. Christine is just amazing at what she does.

Jennifer K

Christine has a fine and special talent as a healer. She was always ahead of the curve with healing methods and treatments. The research and dedication to her work showed with the excellent results her clients enjoyed. She was always my first port of call if my family had any health concerns.

Ciara Browne

Thanks to Christine and her homeopathy treatment, my family and I are in great health. From the age of 10 Christine has worked her magic on me. She has certainly been wonderful to me, always so responsive to any health concerns, and believe me there have been many. I brought my 2 daughters to Christine when they were 6 weeks old. From food intolerances to toothaches and breech babies I can honestly say my family's life is better because of her. I wish her every success with this book. Christine, you deserve it.

Jennifer J

I've been attending Christine for almost 30 years with various ailments which have included digestive issues, hormone imbalance, skin problems and muscular pain. For each problem Christine prescribed homeopathic remedies, many of which she made up from the flower remedies and others from New Vistas which I have to say have worked wonders. Christine has a wealth of knowledge and is unique in her approach to alternative medicine. Due to attending Christine over the years I am now a very healthy 60-year-old.

MY JOURNEY'S END

Today, Sunday 13 August 2023, I am sitting finishing up my story of my life's journey.

And having battled through the diagnosis of my breast cancer through the surgery, chemotherapy and radiotherapy I'm here feeling very well.

I still have a few years ahead on chemotherapy medication to take to keep me cancer free. I still take my homoeopathic remedies which I took all thoughout. From chemotherapy starting I took Bioplasma tissue salts from New Vistas. These I found helped to balance and prevent deficiencies and kept the regular functioning of my body's cells. I also take bone liquescence to keep all my bone tissues strong which is very important when on the hormone therapy post-cancer.

Thirdly, amino acid liquescence helps with repairing tissue, the formation and function of enzymes, food digestion and immune system. I also take PFX for natural pain relief for my hand which has nerve tissue damage.

On Sunday 10 August I visited the lymphedema clinic in Omagh to be told I was in excellent condition. On leaving the clinic I met a client who was waiting for treatment. She gave me a big hug and said only for Jan De Vries 30 years ago doing a seminar at the Killyhevlin Hotel she wouldn't have heard of me. She and her partner had been attending me all those years. She put a smile and a feeling of great contentment and joy in me to know that all these people who have been sending me cards, flowers, visits and been there taking me to all my appointments from January to now have not forgotten me. I continually get text messages, phone calls from them all, and I thank you for your tender care and thoughts all the way.

I hope to continue in some aspect to be of help to them all and that is why I have written this book to be a continued guide and source of help to them all.

AN ACKNOWLEDGMENT

When I opened Nature's Choice in 1995, I wasn't sure if natural health would mean much to people and so I was delighted when Christine Allen walked into the shop within the first few days. Christine was a renowned reflexologist and kinesiologist working within my locality. She had established a busy practice with clients travelling from all over Ireland to avail of her service and she was a well-known advocate for natural health in the area.

To this day Christine continues to draw a huge number of people to her for her knowledge and skill. I believe her to be a gifted healer. She possesses a rare natural instinct when it comes to solving people's health issues and her style and manner in dealing with people ensures that her clients have a clear understanding of how to resolve their health issues.

Christine has amassed a wealth of knowledge on various aspects of natural health throughout her 30 plus years of working within the field. She has moved and progressed with the industry and has kept herself abreast of new skills, new products and new learning. This has been fundamental to her success story.

Christine has helped so many people overcome difficult

health issues. She is acutely aware of the connection between emotional, mental and physical health and understands the importance of holistic health. Christine believes in energy healing and to this end uses her knowledge of homoeopathy and flower essences in particular to help her clients.

Christine has been a great friend of Nature's Choice over the years and we are thrilled to have a close association with her. While Christine and I were probably drawn together by our communal and early interest in natural health, we have become good friends over the years. Christine is honest and generous. I have seen her give, well beyond the course of duty, on too many occasions to remember. Christine is fun, tells a great story and possess a great sense of humour.

Christine's ability to smile and get on with living during ill health has been inspirational. She has set the bar high in how to deal with adversity. It is no surprise to those who know her to learn that she used her "time off work" to write a book. I wish Christine continued good health, a continued successful career in helping and serving others and I wish her every success with her book, so aptly entitled "The Feet I Have Felt".

Nuala Lilley